101 Natural Home Remedies

By

Gene Ashburner

ISBN-13:978-1508789451
ISBN-10:1508789452

Content

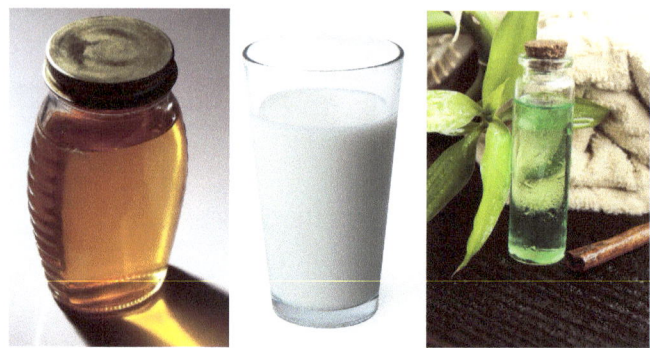

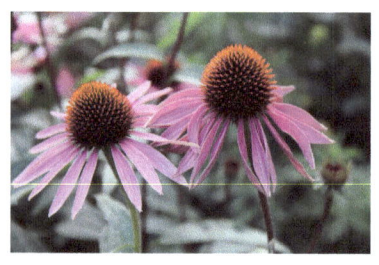

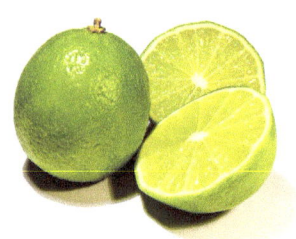

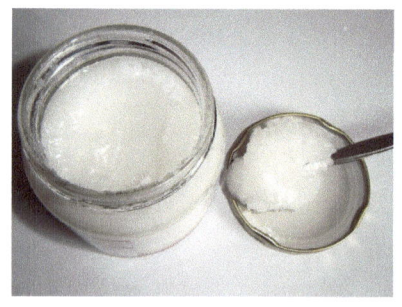

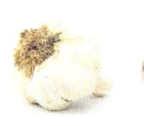

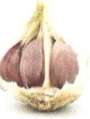

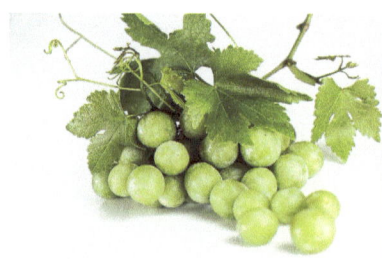

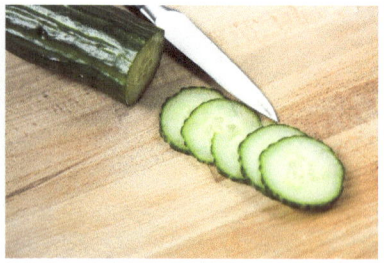

Acid Reflux – Apple Cider Vinegar Remedy

Ingredients

25 ml apple cider vinegar

250 ml water

Method

Combine the apple cider vinegar and water together.

Mix well.

Drink the apple cider mixture 3 times a day.

Acid Reflux - Ginger Remedy

Ingredients

50 g ginger

250 ml water

Method

Combine the ginger and water together.

Mix well.

Drink the ginger mixture after each meal 3 times per day.

Acid Reflux – Herbal Teas

Drink any one of the following herbal teas to reduce acid reflux:

Peppermint tea

Chamomile tea

Ginger tea

Licorice root tea

Catnip tea

Acne – Honey Remedy

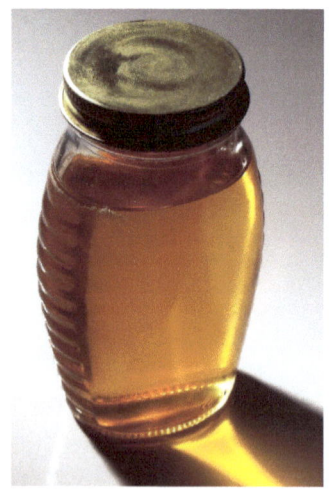

Ingredients

20 ml organic honey

1 apple (peeled, cored and grated)

Method

Combine the honey and apple together.

Mix well.

Apply the paste to the face.

Leave for 10 minutes.

Rinse the face with warm water.

Repeat the procedure twice a week.

Acne – Vinegar Remedy

Ingredients

Distilled white vinegar

Cotton balls

Method

Apply the vinegar to the face and affected acne areas using a cotton ball.

Leave for 5 to 10 minutes.

Rinse off with cool water.

Athletes Foot – Lavender Remedy

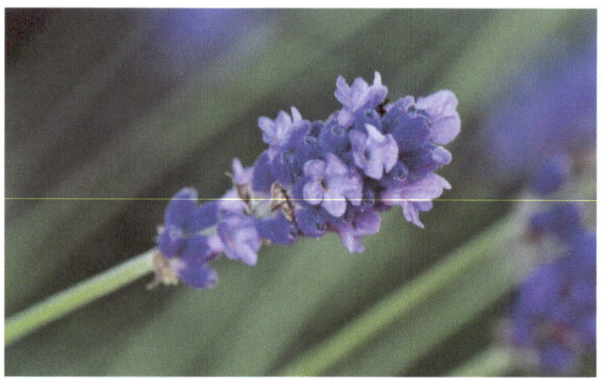

Ingredients

Lavender oil

Alcohol solution

Method

Combine the lavender oil and alcohol solution together.

Mix well.

Soak the feet in the lavender oil and alcohol solution.

Bladder Infections - Cranberry Remedy

Ingredients

Unsweetened cranberry juice

Method

Drink unsweetened cranberry juice daily.

Cranberries contain substances that kill bacteria.

Note:

Do not drink sweetened cranberry juice or cranberry / apple juice as this will aggravate the bladder infection.

Bladder Infections – Yogurt Remedy

Ingredients

250 ml plain yogurt

Method

Eat plain yogurt 4 to 5 times per week.

Blisters - Baby Powder Remedy

Ingredients

Baby powder

Method

Prevent shoes from making blisters on your feet by rubbing baby powder on your feet.

Note:

Keeping your feet from getting sweaty prevents blisters.

Blisters – Listerine Remedy

Ingredients

Few drops Listerine

Method

Apply the Listerine to broken blisters.

The Listerine acts as an antiseptic.

Blisters – Tannic Acid Remedy

Ingredients

10% tannic acid

Method

Apply the tannic acid to the required area of the skin.

Apply twice daily.

Continue this for at least 3 weeks.

Burns – Eucalyptus Oil Remedy

Ingredients

Few drops eucalyptus oil

Method

Apply the oil on the burnt area of skin.

Eucalyptus oil is an extremely potent antiseptic.

Burns - Honey Remedy

Ingredients

Honey

Gauze

Method

Apply pure honey onto a minor burn.

Cover with gauze.

The honey will cool the wound and remove the pain.

Honey also aids fast healing.

Burns – Milk Remedy

Ingredients

Milk

Method

Soak the burned area in the milk for 15 minutes.

You could also apply a cloth soaked in milk to the affected burnt area.

The milk will soothe the burns and promote healing.

Burns - Mustard Remedy

Ingredients

Mustard

Method

Rub mustard onto a minor burn.

It will sting but it reduces pain, blisters and scarring.

Burns - Potato Remedy

Ingredients

Potato slices

Gauze

Method

Place potato slices on the burnt area of skin.

The starch in the potato neutralizes the burn and pain.

The potato starch also prevents scarring.

Cover the potato slices with gauze.

Cankers, Abscesses And Mouth Sores – Salt Remedy

Ingredients

Warm water

Salt

Method

Combine the warm water and salt together.

Mix well.

Rinse the mouth with the salt water solution several times a day.

Constipation – Blackberry Remedy

Ingredients

125 ml distilled water

125 ml blackberries

Method

Combine the distilled water and blackberries together.

Mix well.

Drink the blackberry mixture first thing in the morning.

Constipation - Fig Remedy For Constipation

Ingredients

3 fresh figs

1 banana (peeled and sliced)

12,5 ml honey

250 ml rice dream

Method

Combine the figs, banana slices, honey and rice dream together in a blender.

Blend until smooth.

Drink the Smoothie first thing in the morning and after dinner in the evening.

Cradle Cap - Almond Oil Remedy

Ingredients

Sweet almond oil

Method

Wipe the affected scalp area with sweet almond oil.

Leave the almond oil on for 10 minutes.

Wash the baby's scalp with an organic baby wash or shampoo.

Do not leave the oil on the scalp as this will cause further dryness.

Dental Care – Mouth Wash

Ingredients

Wheat grass (juiced)

Method

Use the wheat grass juice as a mouth wash.

The wheat grass prevents tooth decay.

Dental Care – Teeth Whitening Remedy

Ingredients

6 strawberries

10 ml baking soda

5 ml cream of tartar

250 ml water

Method

Combine the strawberries, baking soda, cream of tartar and water together in a blender.

Blend until smooth.

Apply the puree mixture to the teeth.

Leave overnight.

Repeat the process for a week.

Dental Care – Teeth Whitening Remedy 2

Ingredients

Bicarbonate of soda

Method

Brush the teeth with bicarbonate of soda.

Then brush the teeth with normal toothpaste.

This can be done every 15 days to keep the teeth white.

Depression – Asparagus Remedy

Ingredients

2 g asparagus root (crushed to form a powder)

Method

Take 2 g crushed asparagus root daily to aid with depression.

Depression – Mild Sedative And Calming Agent Lemon Balm Remedy

Ingredients

Lemon balm tea or tincture

Method

Lemon balm can be used as a mild sedative or calming agent when taken in the form of a tea or tincture.

Digestion – Green Tea Remedy

Ingredients

Green tea

Method

Drink a cup of green tea after each meal.

Green tea assists the digestion process and soothes the stomach's sensitive tissue.

Digestion - Peppermint Oil Or Peppermint Leaf Remedy

Use peppermint to treat indigestion, nausea, and abdominal cramps.

Ingredients

250 ml boiling water

10 ml peppermint leave (finely chopped)

Method

Pour the boiling water over the peppermint leaves.

Leave the tea to steep for 10 minutes.

Strain the tea.

Drink the peppermint tea after each meal.

Ear Ache - Swimmers Ear

Ingredients

2 ml ground turmeric

50 ml coconut oil

Method

Combine the turmeric and coconut oil together.

Mix well.

Drops a few drops of the mixture into the affected ear.

Repeat 2-3 times per day until the ear has healed.

Fever Blisters – Cornstarch Remedy

Ingredients

Cornstarch

Water

Method

Combine the cornstarch and water together to form a stiff paste.

Apply the paste to the affected area.

Fever Blisters – Grapefruit Seed Extract Remedy

Ingredients

Few drops grapefruit seed extract

Olive oil

Method

Combine the grapefruit seed extract and olive oil together.

Mix well.

Dab the mixture on the fever blister.

Fever Blisters – St. John's Wort

Ingredients

Few drops St. John's Wort essential oil

Method

Dab the St. John's Wort onto the fever blister.

It soothes, reduces the pain and speeds up the healing process.

Fever Blisters – Teabag Remedy

Ingredients

1 teabag

250 ml boiling water

Method

Steep a teabag in boiling water.

Leave the teabag to cool.

Apply the teabag to the fever blister.

Fever Blisters – Witch Hazel Remedy

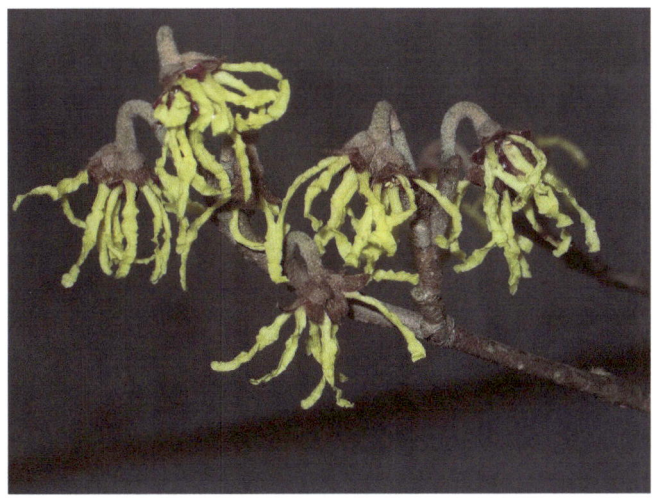

Ingredients

Few drops Witch Hazel

Method

Apply the Witch Hazel to the fever blisters.

Fibroids – Apple Cider Vinegar Remedy

Ingredients

12,5 ml apple cider vinegar

Method

Take 12,5 ml apple cider vinegar 3 times per day.

This may shrink fibroids.

Fibroids – Molasses Remedy

Ingredients

12,5 ml molasses

Method

Take 12,5 ml molasses 3 times per day.

This may shrink fibroids.

Flu, Colds And Sinus - Garlic Remedy

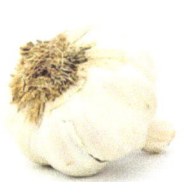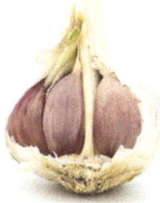

Ingredients

1 clove garlic (peeled)

Method

Place the clove of garlic in the mouth.

Bite down every so-often to release the natural garlic juices.

Replace the clove every 4 hours.

Cold symptoms should be gone within 1 to 2 days.

Flu, Colds And Sinus - Green Onions And Leek Remedy

Ingredients

Leeks

Onions

Method

Eat plenty of leeks and green onions.

These herbs will help fight the cold.

Flu, Colds And Sinus – Lime Remedy

Ingredients

750 ml water

Juice from 5 limes

20 ml honey

Method

Combine the water and lime juice together in a saucepan.

Bring to the boil.

Boil until the mixture has reduced by half.

Remove from the heat.

Add the honey.

Mix well.

Drink the mixture while it is warm.

Flu, Colds And Sinus – Sore Throat Remedy

Ingredients

Lime juice

Method

Drink lime juice to relieve a sore throat.

Flu, Colds And Sinus - Spicy Food Remedy

Ingredients

Spicy foods

Method

Eating spicy foods will open up blocked nasal passages.

Hair – Coconut Dandruff Remedy

Ingredients

Coconut Oil (chilled)

Method

Rub the coconut oil directly onto the scalp.

Leave overnight.

Wash hair with shampoo and warm water.

Hair – Lice Remedy

Ingredients

125 ml coconut shampoo

125 ml Tea Tree oil

Method

Combine the coconut shampoo and Tea Tree oil together.

Mix well.

Rub the shampoo onto the hair.

Leave for 2 hours.

Rinse with warm water.

Comb hair with a metal nit removal comb.

Treat at least 3 more times within the next 2 weeks.

Hair – Lime Dandruff Remedy

Ingredients

Lime juice

Method

Rub lime juice onto the scalp.

Leave for 30 minutes.

Wash out with shampoo and warm water.

Hangover Cure – Banana Smoothie Remedy

Ingredients

4 bananas (peeled, sliced and frozen)

250 ml ice cubes

62,5 ml half and half

Method

Place all the ingredients into a blender.

Blend until smooth.

Drink immediately.

Hangover Prevention – Bifidus Powder Remedy

Ingredients

5 ml Bifidus powder

250 ml water

Method

Combine the Bifidus powder and water together.

Mix well.

Drink the mixture before you go to sleep.

Bifidus powder is a friendly bacteria that detoxifies acetaldehyde which is a by product of alcohol.

This causes the hangover symptoms.

Headaches – Grape Remedy

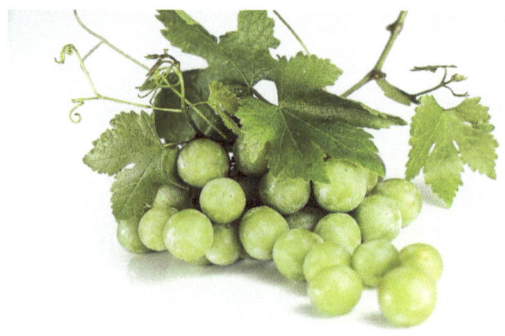

Ingredients

Grape juice or a bowl of grapes

Method

Either eat a bowl of grapes or drink the grape juice.

Headaches – Peppermint Oil Remedy

Ingredients

Few drops peppermint oil

Cotton balls

Method

Place a few drops of peppermint oil onto a cotton ball.

Apply the oil to the forehead.

Take a few minutes to relax and allow the oil to penetrate the skin.

Haemorrhoids – Apple Cider Vinegar Remedy

Ingredients

Apple cider vinegar

Cotton balls

Method

Apply the apple cider vinegar directly onto the affected area using a cotton ball.

The apple cider vinegar behaves as an astringent.

It decreases the actual liquids within the swollen rectal cells.

Haemorrhoids – Cranberry Juice

Ingredients

50 ml raw cranberries (pureed)

Method

Wrap 12,5 ml of pureed cranberries in some cheesecloth

Push it up against the anus and keep it there with some tight underwear.

After an hour or so replace the cranberries with a new batch of cranberries and cloth.

It is high in vitamins and minerals and is effective in treating haemorrhoids since it's an anti-inflammatory and helps encourage regular bowel movements.

Both are essential in getting rid of haemorrhoids.

Haemorrhoids - Fenugreek Seeds

Ingredients

12,5 m fenugreek seeds

Water

250 ml water

20 ml honey

Method

Soak the fenugreek seeds in the water for 5 to 6 hours.

Add the 250 ml water.

Boil the water for 5 minutes.

Add the honey.

Mix well.

Drink the mixture 3 times daily.

High Blood Pressure – Garlic Remedy

Ingredients

Garlic (peeled)

Method

Eat garlic in your food.

Garlic lowers the blood pressure and helps reduce levels of clotting.

High Blood Pressure – Hawthorn Remedy

Ingredients

Hawthorn tea

Method

Drink Hawthorn tea daily.

Hawthorn is known to cause the dilation of the coronary vessels.

It has been used to treat high blood pressure when taken over a period of time.

High Blood Pressure – Potassium And Magnesium Remedy

Potassium and magnesium are vital to the control of elevated blood pressure.

Ingredients

Bananas

Kidney beans

Molasses

Soy

Watermelon

Grapes

Method

Include these food types in the diet.

These foods are considered excellent resources of potassium and magnesium.

Hot Flashes (Flushes) – Coconut Oil Remedy

Ingredients

Coconut oil

Method

Coconut oil is an effective remedy for hot flashes during menopause.

Drink 2 to 3 tablespoons of coconut oil daily.

Insect Bites – Bed Bug Bites

Ingredients

Water

Baking powder

Salt

Method

Combine the water, baking powder and salt together.

Mix well.

Apply the paste to the bed bug bites.

Insect Bites – Bee Sting Remedy

Ingredients

Water

Salt

Method

Wet the area around the bee sting with the water.

Rub salt into the skin.

Insect Bites – Mosquito Bites

Ingredients

Water

Salt

Method

Wet the area around the mosquito bite with water.

Rub salt into the skin.

Insect Repellent – Eucalyptus Remedy

Ingredients

Eucalyptus oil

Method

Eucalyptus oil can be used as an insect repellent.

Rub the eucalyptus oil on all exposed skin areas.

Insect Repellent - Yarrow Remedy

This remedy will repel ticks, mosquitoes, and black flies.

Ingredients

Diluted tincture of yarrow

Method

Apply the tincture on all exposed skin areas.

Menopause – Beet Remedy

Ingredients

60 ml beetroot juice

Method

Drink 60 ml beetroot juice 3 times per day.

Menstruation Relief – Coconut Oil Remedy

Ingredients

Coconut oil

Method

Take coconut oil internally to aid with menstrual pain, cramps and heavy blood flow.

Drink 2 to 3 tablespoons of coconut oil daily.

Menstruation Relief – Ginger Remedy

Ingredients

5 ml ground ginger

250 ml boiling water

Method

Combine the ginger and boiling water together.

Mix well.

Leave to cool.

Drink all at once.

Poison Ivy – Coffee Remedy

Ingredients

125 ml baking soda

Black coffee (enough to form a thick paste with the baking soda)

Method

Combine the baking soda and coffee together to form a thick paste.

Mix well.

Apply the paste onto the rash.

Leave the paste to dry naturally.

Poison Ivy – Salt Water Remedy

Ingredients

Hot water

Salt

Method

Combine the hot water and salt together.

Mix well.

Soak the exposed skin in hot salt water.

This helps stop the poison ivy irritation.

Rheumatism / Arthritis - Alfalfa Remedy

Ingredients

Alfalfa tea

Method

Drink alfalfa tea daily.

Alfalfa herb tea possesses no adverse components and is safe for adults and children.

Rheumatism / Arthritis - Bitter Gourd Remedy

Ingredients

250 ml bitter gourd juice

5 ml honey

Method

Combine the bitter gourd juice and honey together.

Mix well.

Take daily for at least 3 months.

Rheumatism / Arthritis - Celery Remedy

Ingredients

10 drops celery seed extract

250 ml hot water

Method

Combine the celery seed extract and hot water together.

Mix well.

Drink the mixture hot.

Rheumatism / Arthritis - Lemon Juice Remedy

Ingredients

Juice of 3 lemons

Method

Drink the lemon juice daily.

Rheumatism / Arthritis – Potato Remedy

Ingredients

10 ml potato juice

Method

Take 10 ml potato juice before every meal.

Rheumatism / Arthritis – Rhubarb Remedy

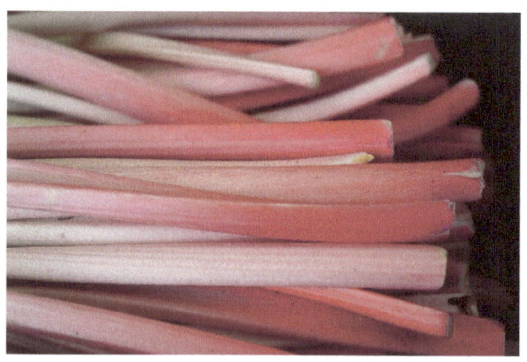

Ingredients

1 rhubarb stalk (mashed)

Sugar

Method

Combine the mashed rhubarb and an equal amount of sugar together.

Mix well.

Take 5 ml of this mixture daily.

Rheumatism / Arthritis - Tea Tree Oil Remedy

Ingredients

18 drops tea tree oil

30 ml almond oil

Method

Combine the tea tree oil and almond oil together.

Mix well.

Pour the mixture into a dark bottle.

Shake before applying.

Apply topically 2 to 4 times per day.

Rheumatism / Arthritis - Tea Tree Oil Remedy 2

Ingredients

3 drops tea tree oil

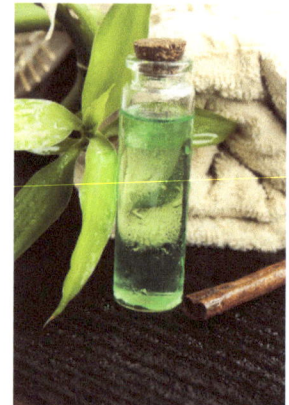

Method

Pour the tea tree oil into a warm bath.

Relax in the warm water.

Rheumatism / Arthritis - Walnut Remedy

Ingredients

6 walnuts (shelled)

Method

Eat the walnuts daily.

Shingles – Aspirin Remedy

Ingredients

2 aspirin tablets (powdered)

25 ml alcohol

Method

Combine the crushed aspirin tablets and alcohol together.

Mix well.

Apply the paste to the affected area.

Shingles - Baking Soda Remedy

Ingredients

Baking soda

Water

Method

Combine baking soda and water together to form a paste.

Mix well.

Apply the solution using a cold compress.

Shingles - Colloidal Powder Remedy

Ingredients

Colloidal powder

Method

Dust the affected area with colloidal powder.

Shingles - Pear Juice Remedy

Ingredients

750 ml pear juice

Method

Drink at least 3 glasses (750 ml) of pear juice per day.

Pears contain antiviral caffeic acid.

Shingles - Vinegar Remedy

Ingredients

125 ml apple cider vinegar

500 ml water

Cotton wool balls

Method

Combine the apple cider vinegar and water together.

Mix well.

Moisten the cotton wool ball with the vinegar mixture and moisten the affected areas using upward movements.

Skin - Black Head Remedy

Ingredients

62,5 ml hot water

5 ml Epsom salt

4 drops iodine

Cotton wool balls

Method

Combine the hot water, Epsom salts and iodine together.

Mix well.

Leave the mixture to cool until lukewarm.

Apply the mixture onto the affected area with a cotton wool ball.

Leave the mixture to dry on the skin.

Remove gently with a clean cloth and warm water.

Skin - Black Head Remedy 2

Ingredients

Ground radish seeds

Water

Method

Combine the radish seeds and water together to form a paste.

Mix well.

Apply the paste onto the affected skin areas.

Leave the paste on the skin to dry.

Wash off with warm water.

Skin - Black Head Remedy 3

Ingredients

Fresh fenugreek leaves (chopped)

Water

Method

Mix the fenugreek leaves with water to form a paste.

Mix well.

Apply the paste on the face every night.

Wash off with warm water in the morning.

Skin – Black Head Remedy 4

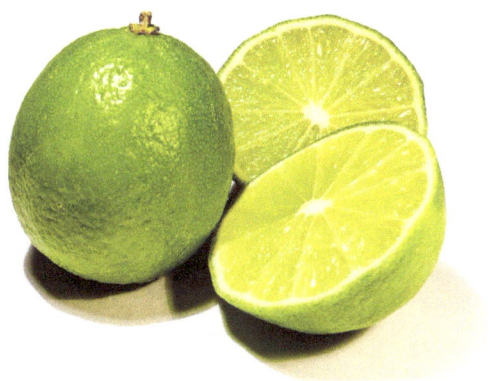

Ingredients

Limejuice

Powdered pomegranate skin (roasted)

Method

Combine the limejuice and powdered pomegranate skin together.

Mix well.

Apply the paste on the face every night.

Wash off with warm water in the morning.

Skin – Black Head Remedy 5

Ingredients

250 ml glycerin soap

125 ml fuller's earth

500 ml almond powder

Boiled water

Method

Combine the glycerin soap, fuller's earth and almond powder together.

Mix well.

Add enough boiled water to make a paste.

Mix well.

Apply the paste to the blackheads.

Leave to dry.

Wash off with warm water.

Skin – Bruises Remedy

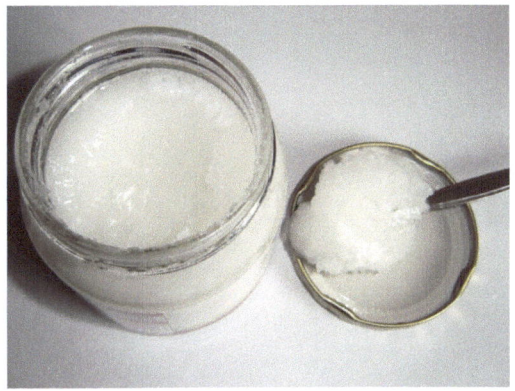

Ingredients

Coconut oil

Method

Coconut oil reduces swelling and redness on bruises.

Apply the coconut oil directly onto the bruise.

Skin – Darkened Elbow Remedy

Ingredients

25 ml lemon juice

25 ml cream

Method

Combine the lemon juice and cream together.

Mix well.

Apply the mixture onto the elbows.

Leave for 30 minutes.

Rinse off with tepid water.

Skin – Oily Skin Lime Remedy

Ingredients

Lime juice

Method

Rub lime juice on the face (especially on the oily T zone).

Lime juice causes the skin pores to contract.

Skin – Pimple Papaya Remedy

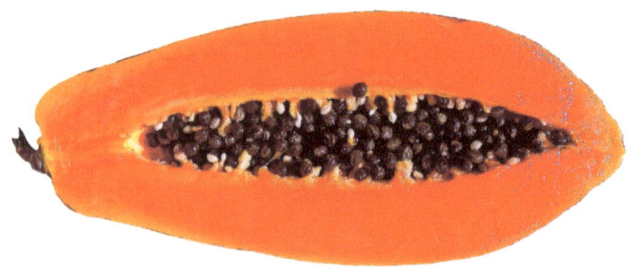

Ingredients

Papaya juice

Method

Apply raw papaya juice, including the skin and seeds onto swelling pimples.

Leave for 15 minutes.

Rinse with warm water.

This will prevent pimples.

Skin – Pimple Tomato Remedy

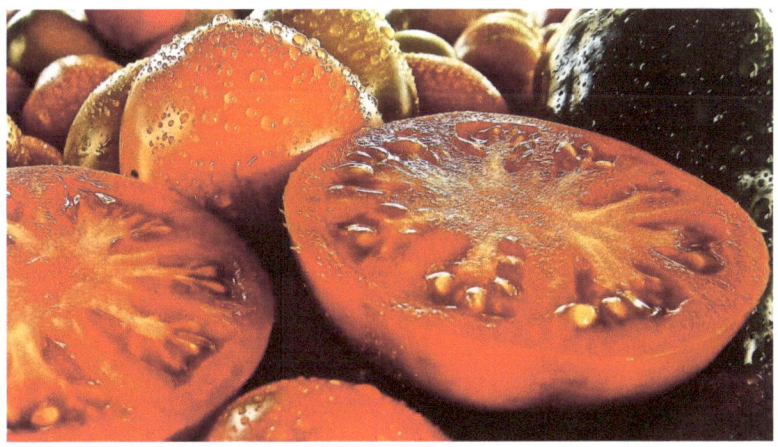

Ingredients

Tomatoes (sliced)

Method

Apply ripe tomatoes pulp on pimples.

Leave for 1 hour.

Rinse off with tepid water.

Skin – Soft Lip Remedy

Ingredients

Lemon juice

Glycerin

Method

Apply glycerin to the lips first.

Apply the lemon juice over the glycerin.

Leave the lemon and glycerin on the lips for 10 minutes.

Wash the mixture off the lips.

Skin – Soft Lip Remedy 2

Ingredients

Almond oil

Method

Apply almond oil onto the lips.

Sneezing – Echinacea Remedy

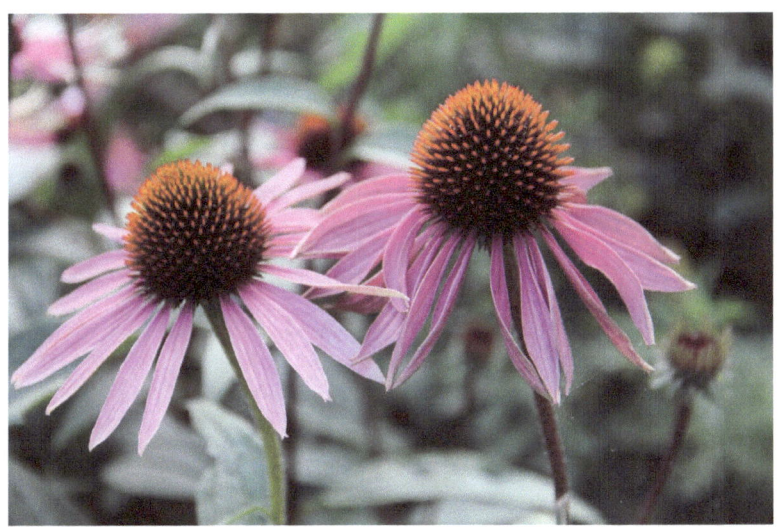

Ingredients

Echinacea tea

Method

Drink Echinacea tea to stop sneezing.

Echinacea is an excellent immunity booster.

Stomach Ulcers - Cayenne Pepper Remedy

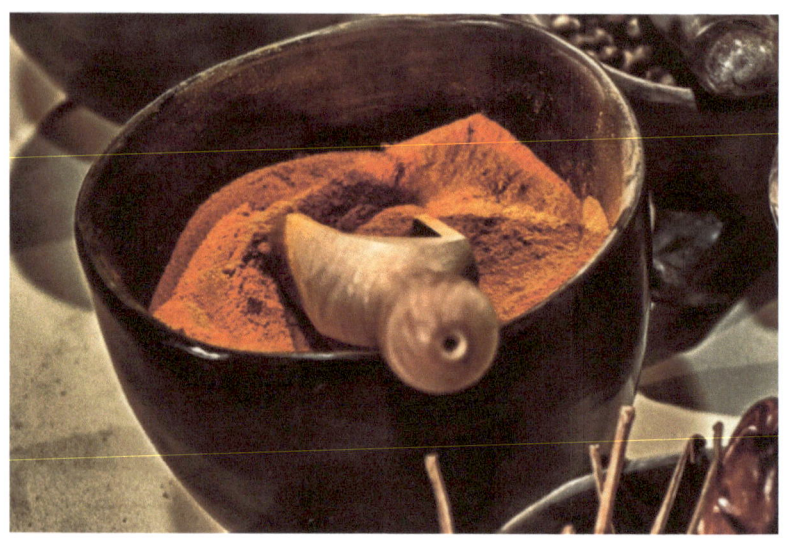

Ingredients

5 ml cayenne pepper

Water

Method

Combine the cayenne pepper and water together.

Mix well.

Drink the mixture.

Cayenne pepper can reduce pain which serves as a local anaesthetic to ulcerated tissue in the stomach.

It also helps to control bleeding in the stomach.

Sun Burn – Baking Soda Remedy

Ingredients

250 ml baking soda

Method

Add the baking soda to the bath water.

Lie and soak in the water.

Sun Burn – Coconut Oil Remedy

Ingredients

Coconut oil

Method

Rub coconut oil onto the affected sun burnt area.

Toe Nail Fungus - Tea Tree Oil Remedy

Ingredients

2 drops tea tree oil

Method

Apply the tea tree oil directly onto the infected toe nails.

Rub the oil above and under the tip of the nail.

Repeat this daily.

Toothache – Clove Oil Remedy

Ingredients

Few drops clove oil

Method

Apply a few drops of clove oil onto the sore tooth.

Clove is an analgesic and will reduce the soreness.

Toothache - Cucumber Remedy

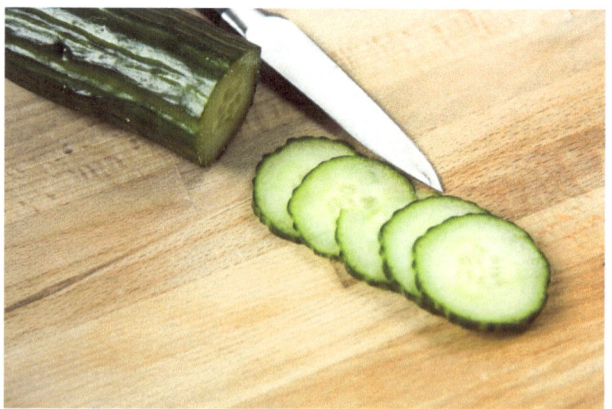

Ingredients

Cucumber

Method

Cut the cucumber into thick slices.

Refrigerate the cucumber slices.

Bite down on the cold cucumber slices.

The cold cucumber slices will sooth the toothache.

Toothache - Iodine Remedy

Ingredients

1 drop Iodine

Method

Place a drop of iodine onto the affected tooth.

Make sure you do not swallow the iodine.

Toothache - Vanilla Extract Remedy

Ingredients

Vanilla extract

Cotton balls

Method

Dab vanilla extract onto the affected tooth using a cotton ball.

The vanilla extract numbs the pain.

Wart Removal - Duct Tape Remedy

Ingredients

> Duct tape
>
> Pumice stone

Method

Place a piece of duct tape over the wart and leave for a week.

The wart will be very soft after the week so now you can scrub the wart off with a pumice stone.

If the wart is not totally gone reapply the duct tape to the wart for another week and continue the process.

Yeast Infections - Tea Tree Oil Remedy

Ingredients

3 or 4 drops Tea Tree Oil

1 Tampon

Olive Oil

Method

Coat the top half of the tampon with olive oil.

Apply the tea tree oil onto the tampon over the olive oil.

Insert the tampon into the vagina.

www.ingramcontent.com/pod-product-compliance
Lightning Source LLC
Chambersburg PA
CBHW050817290526
45792CB00001B/159